Table of Contents

JUICING RECIPES YOUR KIDS WILL LOVE

By: Drew Canole

www.fitlife.tv

Published by Drew Canole
Copyright © 2014, Fitlife TV LLC

ISBN: 1505670098
ISBN-13: 978-1505670097

Passing On the Juice Tradition

A young woman stands in the kitchen of her first home away from home. It's quiet, but her thoughts drown out the silence. This is her kitchen. This is her place. These are her things. While she is excited to be embarking on this adventure into adulthood, she can't help but long for a few more of those carefree days as a child.

Thoughts of family meals rush through her mind, and she quickly locates an unpacked box that holds something very special to her. She reaches in and pulls out a small container. What does it hold?

It is a gift from her mother, which was a gift from her mother. A collection of cards, carefully handwritten, representing generations of memories... they are recipes.

Sharing is Caring

If you are part of the FitLife community, you've likely heard me talk about sharing your healthy lifestyle with others. This knowledge is just too important, and tasty, to keep to ourselves! For those who are raising young children, your own families are the perfect place to start. In fact, it's probably the reason that you're reading this book.

Sharing your juicing adventure with your children may be easy at times and rather challenging at others. Depending on their ages, their responses could be as varied as the foods you are hoping they'll love. If yours are not convinced, do not give up hope. We will be discussing in a later chapter how you can define their reasons, their "why," for taking a chance on a new food.

You will also discover how you can facilitate a change in how food tastes to your child. Yes, you CAN convince those little taste buds that they would rather have a fresh vegetable over a French fry! Don't believe me? Read on!

What's Eating Your Kids?

We cannot protect them from everything out there, but we can give them a better chance at winning the fight against common childhood ailments. How many times have you heard from fellow parents that a "bug" was running its course through the whole family?

It causes missed days from school, missed days from work (or miserable days AT work) and even missed opportunities for fun family activities. Life goes on, so when illness catches up with us, it's easy to reach into the medicine cabinet for a little help.

But there is a better way (you knew I was going to say that)! Actually, there are two. The first is prevention. Not just an ounce... but a cup! Whole foods have the unmatched power to safely and efficiently raise the shields on each and every cell in your child's body, making them stronger and less susceptible to invasion by little "bully bugs." The second is a healthier, more natural way to fight off what does take hold.

"Let food be thy medicine and medicine be thy food."

- Hippocrates

Kids' Common Ailments

The most effective and efficient way to defend your child's overall health is by regular juicing, preferably every day. By providing a consistent intake of health giving nutrients, you can help your child avoid common ailments such as colds, flu, sore throats, stomachaches and bugs, headaches... and even allergies. Juicing may also help alleviate psychological "aches" such as anxiety, depression and mood swings.

We are excited to provide some basic juice recipes, which will help you win the fight for your child's health. You will find information on the nutrients included through the juice's ingredients, as well as common illnesses that those nutrients may help clear up.

Keep in mind, I am not a doctor, but I am passionate about sharing what I have learned over the years working with clients and doing hours of research. What I share here is not meant to be a substitute for the care and attention of a pediatrician, but a great way to ensure you don't have to visit them as often!

To Wake Them Up, Juice Them Up!

Is your son or daughter struggling to get through the day? Are they tired and can't seem to find enough energy to keep up with the demands of being a teenager? There is a lot of pressure put on our young population, which can easily turn into physical, mental and emotional exhaustion. They need the right kind of fuel... the kind that will energize their physical body and bring them out of the fog into a state of mental clarity.

But first, you need to know that one of the most important factors in bringing your sluggish child up to speed is to slow them all the way down - to sleep. To get the most out of each day, they need to get the most out of each night.

You will get some more tips in just a bit on how you can help your children catch a great night's sleep for optimal health, along with the next most important factor... water. Believe it or not, water has the ability to give your child more energy than anything they can buy from the store that claims it can do the same thing.

The part we have the most fun with is the nutrition blast we get from juicing! There's a reason that fruits and vegetables are so colorful and vibrant... they are full of life! They are packed with energy.

I look at the variety of whole foods and see energy and healing in the colors themselves. Red, blue, yellow, green, purple, orange... they all have so much to offer. Would you agree?

Focusing Their Energy

If your kids aren't the sleepy kind, you might be thinking: "Do I really want my kids to have MORE energy?" My answer to that is...Yes and No! Being energetic is in almost every kid's job description, but let's take a look at what is creating this energy.

Andy is nine years old. He starts the day in high gear and stays that way until he falls asleep, after an exhausting effort by his parents. His favorite foods consist of refined grains (cereals, pasta, baked not-so-goods), sugars (candy, ice cream, sugary drinks), fast food (fries, burgers, pizza, chicken nuggets) with few fruits and vegetables.

He is difficult to control at home, and school is a challenge because he won't sit still. The teacher has mentioned having him tested for Attention Deficit Hyperactivity Disorder. Mom's heart is breaking, because she wants everyone to see how sweet, helpful, and kind Andy is when he isn't running on full tilt. Dad refuses to accept a diagnosis, thinking that the kid just needs a little more discipline. No, he doesn't need more of that kind of "energy."

As an adult, what happens when you drink coffee or soda, to help wake you up in the morning or keep you going in the afternoon? You have an initial rise in energy and you feel you are better able to function, even though you crash not long thereafter. What happens to a child, who is already programmed to be on-the-go, when he consumes artificial sources of energy? His body goes into a frenzy due to sugar and preservative overload, exhausting everyone around him. These man-made "foods" actually act like a drug in those little bodies and brains.

What if we could give Andy some real energy that would help him gain control of his thoughts and actions? This is the kind of focused energy that kids today need, more than ever. Real, living, whole foods, eaten as part of a healthy meal or juiced, will give Andy what he needs to let his true personality come to life.

Your Why, Their Why... Y-Y-Y

You have good reasons for wanting your children to consume healthy, whole foods. You know the benefits that await them at the bottom of each delicious glass of juice. But your little ones also need big reasons for doing things that might not sound like a lot of fun at first.

One mom emailed me recently and told me a story about broccoli. She mentioned to her young son that she was steaming some broccoli for dinner that night, and Dad immediately said "Ew!" Now, I'm not an expert in the field of child psychology, but I'm pretty confident that this isn't the best approach. So what can we do?

Y is for Yummy!

To get kids interested in eating what they should, they have to want to do it. How do you get them to want to eat healthy? Stop telling them it's healthy, and start telling them it's YUMMY! Help them discover that color has taste. Make a game out of finding out what red tastes like, what yellow tastes like... and yes, what green tastes like, too!

The recipes in this book will show you how to begin pairing foods together so that the ones usually rejected will be accepted more easily, with your kids asking for more!

Y is for You

Children of all ages will take an interest in what you are doing, because they love being WITH YOU. They may not know how to express it, but in their hearts what they want most is your time. You have an opportunity to share healthy lifestyle choices with your child by spending time with them and showing them how to do it.

Young children love to put pieces into the juicer to see what comes out. Even if they are shy about trying the juice at first, curiosity will eventually win them over. In the meantime, they'll have fun hanging out with you. And you'll have fun, too.

Y is for Yearning

Depending on their age, all kids want something: to be as smart as another kid in their class at school, to earn a place on the ball team, to have friends. All of these lead to acceptance... from teachers and coaches, from peers, and from you. What does this have to do with juicing? Quite a lot!

When a child's brain is charged up with the fuel he needs, he will be able to focus better in class and learn new concepts more easily.

When a child's body is loaded with healthy energy from life-giving foods that repair and build, she will perform better on the ball field.

When children FEEL better, they are happier, they are more confident, they are better friends to others, and others will want to be around them.

Teens also will be interested to know that eating and juicing nutritionally dense foods will help keep their skin clear... definitely something that they want!

Juice Plus Seven

Giving health-packed foods to young bodies and minds is the cornerstone of a fruitful life (a "vegeta-ful" one, too!). To build on this solid nutritional foundation, several additional factors are essential to the development of happy and healthy futures. I regularly address some of these concepts with members of the FitLife community.

#1... Keep The Sleep

According to the American Psychological Association, "69 percent of children experience one or more sleep problems a few nights or more during a week." When a child does not get enough rest, he may show signs of irritability, problems concentrating in school, an increased susceptibility to illness and risk of serious health problems later in life.

Depending on their age, children need anywhere from 10-12 hours per night for toddlers, to 8-9 hours per night for teens. These are general guidelines, as some individuals may need more based on their own health profile.

Here are some tips to help ensure a healthy night's rest:

1. As much as possible, keep your children on the same sleep/wake schedule from one day to the next, including weekends.
2. Be sure that they are exercising regularly.
3. Avoid electronic stimulation for at least an hour before bedtime.
4. Keep the last meal of the day light, and save the fruits for earlier in the day since they contain natural sugars.
5. Try to avoid over-scheduling them; give them time to wind down.
6. Enjoy a delicious nighttime juice, found in this book's recipes.

#2... Let Them Play

You've probably noticed how quickly time passes... and if you blink, your kids aren't little anymore. Lately it seems that our society wants them to act like little adults, rather than allowing them to be children and simply play. It turns out that it's more important than one might think.

As stated by the American Academy of Pediatrics: "Play is essential to development because it contributes to the cognitive, physical, social, and emotional well-being of children and youth. Play also offers an ideal opportunity for parents to engage fully with their children."

As we focus on academics and enrichment opportunities, we should also make a deliberate effort to allow children to engage in free child-centered play. For the little ones, have fun with play food sets of fruits and vegetables and see what kind of new juice recipes come out of that toy kitchen. If you're brave enough, taste test them!

#3... Rock The Routines

All children need some sort of routine in their lives, some more than others. They need to know what to expect, because it helps give them a sense of stability and control. Sit down with your child or children and, depending on their age, discuss what they think is most important at both the start and end of each day.

Then, stick with the plan as much as you can. Keep the list short and simple. Creating this habit early on in their lives will have a profound effect on their happiness and productivity as they grow older.

Whether you have time to sit down to a family breakfast or are rushing out the door each morning, spending even a small amount of time observing rituals will help start the day on firm footing. Some ideas for the morning include: spend 5-10 minutes reading or have devotional time with your children, have music playing, spend a few minutes talking about what will be happening that day, and talk about what each of you is grateful for.

Don't forget to add a nutritious morning juice as a rock solid foundation to each day! You'll find more great breakfast ideas in the recipes section.

Bedtime can also be stressful if children don't know what to expect. To calm things down, include just a few simple routines which will mark the end of the day and give you some cozy cuddle time with your family.

Reading before bed is one of the #1 ways to relax (for "kids" of all ages), listen to soothing music, allow enough time for a quiet board game or puzzle... or even journal together, which could include writing down their favorite events of the day, or they can draw simple pictures in the journal if they are young.

And always spend time helping them to recognize their blessings. Rituals like this go beyond the usual list of teeth brushing and changing into pajamas, and can make such an impact on your child's daily life and future.

#4... Model A Gratitude Attitude

I appreciate you. I love that you are taking steps to ensure that your family is healthy and happy, and all of us at FitLife feel blessed to be in that together with you. You are a big part of why I wake up every morning feeling grateful to be doing the work that I am.

It wouldn't be worth it if I didn't see amazing transformations every day, with people pushing through difficult circumstances to reach their goals of renewed health and vitality.

What are you grateful for? What are your children grateful for? Many people gather with family one day per year to give thanks for all of the good things that have happened in their lives over the preceding months.

Let me propose a radical idea: that we very purposefully take time out of every morning, every single day of the year, to start our day with gratitude in our minds and hearts. Before your feet hit the floor, take a few minutes to be thankful. You may not have much in the way of material things, but you have another day. Even difficult situations and experiences are an opportunity for us to grow and be thankful.

As you wake your child, sit with her and help her think of how much she is blessed. This is definitely one habit that will make your child's heart soar. And it's also another way that you can bond with your children.

What a special time this could be, that your child will always appreciate as he/she grows older. Challenge yourself and your child to say "thank you" to at least one person each day. You'll be amazed at how this changes your outlook on life, and what it will do for your child's mindset, now and in the future. Powerful!

#5... Give Them An Affirmation Education

Now that you have your kids feeling grateful, let's stack some more positivity into their minds before they venture out into the day. If you're unfamiliar with how affirmations work, you can visit us online at FitLife.tv to learn more about how to set them as a habit in your own life. For now, here's what you need to know to help your kids, starting today.

From a very early age, we tend to adopt the belief systems of those who take care of us and teach us about how the world works. Even children teach each other in social settings and at school, and that's not always a good thing.

What might be true for others may not be true for your child, but that won't stop him from believing what he hears. It's important, then, that you teach him how to adopt a set of positive beliefs so that what isn't true doesn't have a lasting negative effect on his emotions and mindset.

Here are several examples of positive affirmations for young children: I am loved. Learning new things at home and at school are fun for me. I love being healthy. I am creative and have a great imagination. I am forgiving and kind to others who make mistakes.

I make mistakes, too, but I learn from them to make myself a better person. I have friends who like spending time with me. I am helpful to my parents and teachers. Include affirmations as part of the morning routine to set the day off right! It need only take a few short minutes but will follow your child throughout the day.

#6... Put Your Kids In Motion

If your kids spend most of their time sitting, you have to get them out of the chair. This isn't breaking news. But sometimes it's hard to accomplish, since sedentary activities seem to be dominating children's lives lately, which even in the elementary grades includes sitting for hours each day at school.

Set a reasonable amount of time for them to play with their electronic devices, spend time online, or watch a short television program... but when time is up, it's up and on their feet! If it helps, you can even set a timer so there's no fuss about when activities are due to change. This is especially helpful for the little ones.

Team sports are a fantastic way to keep your kids moving. The range of benefits from team play is so plentiful that it would fill an entire book on its own! Even exercise at home can easily satisfy the cravings for movement by those young bodies and minds.

Bike rides, walks, time at the park or playground with the family are all great ways to spend time together while also getting some fresh air and sunshine. And don't discount the effects of just being on their feet... like standing next to the counter putting yummy veggies in the juicer. And think about this: once your kids get juicing, they may just lose interest in sitting around so much!

#7... Juice Them Up, Water Them Down

As much as your kids will love their juice, it's not a replacement for water. A healthy and life-giving menu includes plenty of both. Our bodies are made up of 75% water and cannot function for long without it. I cannot stress enough the importance of drinking enough water. In addition to leaving their bodies vulnerable to communicable disease, chronic dehydration is a common reason for feeling run-down and fatigued, which makes for cranky kids who have a hard time focusing at school or engaging with the family at home.

"Water is the driving force in nature."
- Leonardo da Vinci

Be sure that you are getting your water from a good source. If an in-home purifier or ionizer is accessible for you, I recommend it. You can also purchase alkaline water. At the very least, be sure you are filtering your water in some form. Even the best quality water is a tough sell for a lot of kids and teens. How do you encourage them to take the glass?

In the recipes section, we've given you some creative ways to serve water that your kids will love. You won't have to, or want to, buy that expensive (and sugary) vitamin water anymore once they've tried these!

Little Buds

Children look to the adults in their life for protection, guidance and inspiration. Everything that they see you do or hear you say will stick with them as they grow and develop their belief sets. This is especially true regarding food choices. They'll believe you when you say a type of food is okay, especially if it tastes good! But what makes certain foods taste good? It depends a lot on where you live!

Compare the standard American diet (SAD, for a reason!) to that of other cultures and small communities throughout the world. In the United States, and increasingly other countries as they adopt the same standards, there is an "anything goes" mentality. Well, almost. Most of the citizens of the United States and Europe will recoil at the thought of eating an insect, while many families across Asia, Africa and Latin America keep them on the menu as traditional staple.

The same people who will gladly eat a protein packed, juicy insect would probably think other people are crazy for eating a chicken nugget (pink slime, anyone?). While kids in small farming communities grow up eating what they grow themselves, kids in and near large cities often start eating fries and gulping down sugar-laden, processed juices before they learn to walk... and many pediatricians see nothing wrong with that.

The truth is that your kids will adopt the tastes to which they are exposed. Your children will learn to prefer the foods that you consistently provide for them, and it starts before they are born. But if your baby is not a baby anymore and unhealthy foods have already been introduced, don't worry. You CAN change their taste preferences. I help adults do this very thing every day. To learn more about how you can change your taste, pick up my e-book titled *Train Your Taste To Trim Your Waist* - available on Amazon.

With adults, I recommend starting with the "Alpha Reset" juice fast protocol. Think of it this way: In finer restaurants, you'll often be served a palate cleanser between or as one of the lighter courses. The reason for this is that you have a greater appreciation for varying flavors if you clear your senses before going on to the next.

The juice fast accomplishes this in its own way. It clears out the craving for sweets and unhealthy fats, and gives your taste buds the opportunity to appreciate the flavors in fruits and vegetables as never before. People who typically avoid leafy greens find themselves starting to actually crave them.

However, I don't recommend juice fasting for children. You can still clear their palate in a more gradual way. Instead of taking their favorite foods out of their diet in a way that would be very abrupt and upsetting for the younger ones, my suggestion is to slowly add in more healthy options as time passes.

You may also find that slightly changing the recipes is a way that you can increase the nutritional value of a meal without a lot of fuss. Your children should start to become accustomed to the new additions without missing the ones you've casually dropped along the way.

A good place to start is with simple fresh juices, to replace the unrecognizable ones bought in the store in a box or jug. Just switch out the orange juice, the apple juice, even the grape juice if that's what your child likes. Keep it simple. In the journey to introduce a picky young eater to the delicious world of juicing, you may find yourself wanting to break a few rules along the way. One of those rules has to do with juicing fruits.

You'll notice that I mostly advocate for juicing vegetables. There's a reason for that. Fruits, while you can certainly juice them, are still very high in natural sugar content and are better eaten whole or blended.

The body will use the fiber in the fruits to slow absorption and aid in digestion, something that you don't get when juicing them. Even with this, there is still a lot of confusion surrounding the question of whether or not it is okay to mix fruits and vegetables when juicing. The answer is that usually it's better not to.

The goal of clearing the palate and changing taste preferences is jeopardized if we trade one sweet taste for another. So while you may find that the only way to include a vegetable in juice for a young one is to slip it in under the sweet taste of multiple fruits, your child may experience gas and bloating as a result of the body's difficulty in properly digesting them together, and this goes for smoothies, too.

There is an exception, however, with apples and pears. These are easily paired with vegetables to help mask the taste of greens until your child is used to them. Lemons are also a fantastic addition.

One of the best fruit and vegetable mixed juices to start with is simply a couple of apples and a small handful of spinach. You can start with a sweeter variety of apple and work your way to the greener and less sweet tasting ones, like Granny Smith, as your child's preference changes.

The spinach will make the juice green, so if your child has an inexplicable aversion to that color (a common obstacle), one mom's solution is to put his juice in a solid plastic cup with a straw. Make it a silly straw for added fun!

There are parents out there who started their children early by juicing vegetables without the added sweet taste of fruits. I applaud your efforts! If you're a parent who didn't know until your children were older how important juicing is for them, it's okay.

If it's not too late for an adult to change their taste and their health along with it, it is certainly not too late for a child. Take your time, don't try to push the greens too quickly if your kids don't accept them at first, and make it fun!

Imagine This...

The young woman looks at the new juicer sitting on her kitchen counter... a housewarming gift from her parents. She checks the container for a special recipe that reminds her of home, and gathers the ingredients. A family tradition has been passed down... one that promises health and vitality for generations to come.

PART TWO:

Flavored Water

Basic Juicing Tips

Juice Recipes

Juice Builders

Top 5 Juicing Add-Ons

Smoothies

Flavored Water

As you begin to experiment with new recipes and combinations, start with less added and increase to your personal taste. Have fun with your favorite ingredients, and mix it up each day! You can first crush some of the ingredients, and then add slices for visual appeal while entertaining guests. Crushing or twisting fruits or herbs will make the flavor more intense.

Once you are done creating your water recipe, cover and refrigerate for a couple of hours and consume within 1-2 days. You can store your mixed water at room temperature, but not for extended periods of time since the fruit will begin to ferment. The following three recipes were featured on an episode of Saturday Strategy. Enjoy!

Blackberry + Ginger + Lime

Mash about ½ cup of blackberries and drop another ½ cup into about 4 cups of water. Drop in a ginger knuckle (you could grate it, as well), and squeeze ½ of a lime, dropping it in once squeezed. Refrigerate. This recipe is full of antioxidants, helps with digestion, will help to keep your skin healthy, helps with mental clarity and alkalizes your body.

Mint + Raspberry + Strawberry

Drop a small handful of mint leaves into your water first. Next, from about a cup's worth, add some whole raspberries to make it look irresistible, and then crush the rest and add. Next, crush in a handful of strawberries and chill. This recipe is good for congestion, fighting viruses, is full of antioxidants and helps boost cognitive function.

Lemon + Lime + Cucumber

Start by adding about ½ cucumber thinly sliced, followed by ½ each of a lemon and lime, also sliced. That's it! This recipe is perfect for summer months because it cools you down. It alkalizes your body and through its anti-aging properties helps keep you moms out there looking young and vibrant!

More Ingredient Ideas:

There are so many possible combinations that we could share with you, but it will ultimately come down to what flavors you like. Pick your child's favorites, combine them, and then keep the ones that work. Write down the recipes, save them in a special place like a little box, and share them with the community.

I would love to hear where your creativity takes you! Following is a list of the most commonly used fruits, vegetables and extras to help make your water taste exciting and fresh.

Fruits:

Apple, Blackberry, Blueberries, Cantaloupe, Cranberries, Grapefruit, Grapes, Honeydew Melon, Kiwi, Lemon, Lime, Mango Pit, Orange, Pineapple, Raspberry, Strawberry, Watermelon

Vegetables:

Celery, Cucumber, Radish

Herbs & Spices:

Basil, Cilantro, Cinnamon, Ginger, Peppermint, Rosemary, Spearmint, Thyme

Basic Juicing Tips

If your family hasn't included juicing as part of its lifestyle until now, you may need some very simple juice "recipes" to start with until the concept is more easily accepted. There is a lot of flavor in simple juices, and you don't always need to add 5 or more ingredients to make it special. As you introduce these fresh juices, keep the following points in mind:

Serve sweet fruit / fruit juices in the morning while those little tummies are still empty. Fruits should be consumed by themselves and not with any other food.

It's also best not to mix multiple fruits in the same juice or smoothie. Delicious? Yes! But, by mixing many fruits you are increasing the amount of sugar consumed all at once. Through juicing, you are removing the fiber. Fiber slows absorption and helps the body process the sugar in a much healthier way.

As you are introducing the juicing lifestyle to young children, offer only about 6-8 ounces at a time to keep their tummies happy with the change.

Offer less if the juice is made up of sweet fruits. Serve more over time as you switch to more vegetables.

Add water to fruit juices to significantly reduce the sugar rush and reduce the sweet, addictive taste. It's best to do this from the very start of your juicing adventure, but as always, start where you are!

Basic and recognizable vegetable juices, like the ones listed below, may be the best way to introduce veggie juice to kids of any age. I understand that you may feel inclined to include a variety of fruits as you are starting out because you want them to love their juice. But, keep the amounts very low while using fruits.

Over time, adjust the amount of fruit juices that you serve in favor of more vegetables. If you do this gradually, not only will your kids not notice, but they'll begin to accept and even crave the less sugary taste.

Always choose organic produce, when available.

Experiment. Have FUN!

Orange Juice

Sweet fruits like oranges are best eaten alone and with teeth, but if you have an O.J. lover in your house, the taste of freshly juiced oranges will win over anything you'll find on the grocery store shelf. For a sweet treat in the morning, offer orange juice on its own.

Nutrition:

Oranges are highest in Vitamin C, Vitamin A, calcium, and iron.

Health Benefits:

- Helps fight against constipation.
- Wins the war on viral infections.
- Boosts the immune system to stop sniffles and sneezes from sneaking up on you.

Storage:

Keep oranges for up to a week at room temperature, and up to a month in the refrigerator.

Tip:

Citrus juices should be consumed only in moderation, since high amounts can cause the body to lose calcium.

Did You Know?

* The orange blossom is the state flower of Florida.
* Brazil produces the most oranges each year, followed by the United States.
* Navel oranges are named this way because of the extra growth at the top, which resembles a human navel. Call it "Belly Button Juice" for a giggle.

Orange + Apple

Nearly everyone has heard the old adage "An apple a day keeps the doctor away."

Add oranges and juice them together, and you have a powerful weapon against the common viruses that plague our young population. Enjoy this delicious duo for its antiviral properties.

Orange + Carrot

Kids love orange juice. Kids love carrot juice. Put them together and watch what happens. It's an orange delight that your kids will come back to again and again.

Orange + Pineapple + Ginger

Kick it up a notch for an extra burst of energy with this nutrient packed and sweet tasting juice recipe. Go easy on the amount of ginger at first, and increase to about ¼ - ½ inch for every eight ounces of juice, depending on preference.

Orange + Apple + Pear + Lemon

Tackle aches and pains with a glass of this sweet combination. To minimize the sour taste of the lemon for little ones, peel it first and use only about ¼ of a small fruit.

Orange + Apple + Cucumber + Celery + Red Bell Pepper + Lemon + Spinach

Fan Favorite!

Good health has never tasted so good with recipes like this one! Kids agree! This recipe will yield more volume with the water based cucumber and celery on the menu. You can either reduce the amount of other ingredients for a smaller serving, or join your young one with your own fresh glass of yum. Cheers!

Grapefruit Juice

Commonly found on breakfast tables, it might be slightly bitter for young taste buds. Use a bit of stevia to sweeten it up. The pink or red varieties are naturally a bit sweeter, so those might be more eagerly accepted at first.

Peel off the skin of the fruit, but leave as much of the albedo (the white flesh just under the skin) intact when serving this fruit whole.

Nutrition:

Grapefruits are high in Vitamins C, A, B1 and B5, and are a good source of potassium.

Health Benefits:

- Grapefruit juice will help alkalize the body.
- Prevents colds from taking hold.
- Helps reduce the risk of diabetes
- Helps with sore throats, soothe coughs, and reducing fever.
- Helps get little ones to sleep at night if they are having trouble.

Storage:

Grapefruits are slightly juicier when at room temperature. Store them on the counter for up to a week, or in the refrigerator for 2-3 weeks.

Tip:

A word of caution with grapefruits: If your child is currently taking synthetic medication, you should avoid grapefruit juice. It will interact with the potency of the medications. As always, consult with your child's doctor before making any changes to their diet, as they will know best how to proceed based on your child's unique health profile.

Did You Know?

Grapefruits come in red, white and pink. The darker the color, the sweeter it is.

Grapefruit + Lemon + Honey

In addition to all of the benefits of grapefruits and lemons, this combination is useful for waking up those groggy little ones in the morning. Juice equal parts of grapefruit and lemon, and add a little bit of honey to sweeten.

Apple Juice

This is a favorite for toddlers just about everywhere. Rather than handing them a little box with a straw, let them experience what apple juice REALLY tastes like! You can start with the sweeter red varieties and work your way to the green ones which typically have less natural sugar packed within.

Nutrition:

Vitamins A, C, E, B6, riboflavin, thiamin, potassium, calcium and phosphorus.

Health Benefits:

- When eaten whole, the apple's pectin will aid in digestion.
- Helps build and maintain strong bones.
- May help reduce symptoms for children with asthma.
- Helps to strengthen the immune system.
- Add cayenne pepper to apple juice to help with sore throat and prevent strep.

Storage:

In the coolest part of the fridge, most varieties of apple can be stored for up to two weeks.

Tips:

* Add water to apple juice to reduce the sweetness.
* Juice apples with the peel but without the seeds since they are toxic when crushed, and small children may be at greater risk of having a reaction.
* Add apples to green juices to help mask the bitter taste of the leafy greens.

Did You Know?

There are over 7,500 different kinds of apple! When cut on the width, the center of an apple resembles a five-point star.

Apple + Cranberry

Many of us are familiar with the popular red cranberry apple juice sold in stores. Juicing fresh apples and cranberries together brings that taste of these two amazing flavors to the next level - a WOW factor for the senses!

Not only does it taste great, but it also supports the immune system. The amount of cranberries you use will depend on taste preference, but you can start out with a couple of apples and ½ cup of cranberries.

Apple + Spinach

Fan Favorite!

Once your child is happy with his apple juice, try adding a small amount of spinach. I love this pairing for its mild taste and that it is a low-sugar, nutritious way to introduce green juicing to young ones. The juice combination is not overly sweet tasting and though a fruit, apple combines nicely with baby spinach and other vegetables for taste and proper digestion.

Start with two apples and a handful of spinach. Increase the amount of each for older children or as younger ones become accustomed to juicing.

Apple + Carrot + Red Chard

Fan Favorite!

This is a sweet way to introduce a new leafy green to the menu. You can use red chard, or have fun with the different colors of Rainbow Chard, a mixture of different chard varieties.

If you're not sure about chard being accepted by children, you'll be surprised to know that this combination was provided by a fan... and her kids love it!

Apple + Lemon + Ginger

Sniffling? Sneezing? Coughing? Juice up this combination for cold relief. Great for kids and adults alike! Enjoy this recipe on a regular basis to prevent illness. Use a sweeter red apple for kids until they can enjoy the taste of the lemon and ginger with a green apple.

"Stomach Soother"
Apple + Carrot + Cabbage + Ginger

Don't let a tummy ache disrupt another school day (sorry, kids). Cabbage is great at soothing the stomach and helping with indigestion. The sweet apple and carrots make this a delicious remedy that may have them claiming a belly ache just to get it!

"Super Juice"

Fan Favorite!

Start with cucumber as a base since it has a high water content. Apple and carrot will sweeten it up, and your kids will barely notice the taste of kale. Start with one leaf and adjust the amount when they ask for more. Kid-approved!

1. Base veggies: **Cucumber**
2. Sweeteners: **Apple + Carrot**
3. Greens: **Kale**

Pear Juice

While the fiber content of pears make them a perfect snack or for adding to smoothies, juiced pears also create a delightful sweet treat! They can be a source of fun and discovery, too, since they come in so many different varieties and several colors.

Nutrition:

Pears contain Vitamins C and A, B complex vitamins, copper, iron, potassium, manganese, magnesium, and antioxidants.

Health Benefits:

- Pear juice will cool you down during the hot summer days.
- Helps alleviate a sore throat.
- Contains antioxidants, which will head off that cold that may be knocking at the door.
- Pears are an excellent anti-inflammatory food to help with aches and pains.
- A mild diuretic which will alleviate constipation.

- A big glass of fresh pear juice is also one of the tastiest ways to help reduce a fever. No more medicine yuck faces!

Storage:

Allow pears to ripen at room temperature, and then store in the refrigerator for 2-3 days.

Tip:

Pears can be juiced with the peel on, but with the seeds removed. Water down the sweeter varieties if serving as a single juice. Pears are a common and delicious way to sweeten up green juices and smoothies.

Did You Know?

This fruit ripens from the inside out; consume when the neck becomes soft.

Pear + Kiwi

Juice up their healthy energy with this simple but powerful combination. In addition to the many benefits of pear, adding kiwi will kick up the Vitamins C, K, and E. You don't have to peel kiwifruit before juicing, but note that the skin has a bitter taste and might not be easily accepted by little taste buds.

Pear + Apple + Cinnamon

Many kids love the apple and cinnamon combination in foods such as oatmeal. Bring that fun and festive flavor to life in a juice with pear to help sweeten it up. Really, really good! The cinnamon has also been shown to have antiviral properties, so pull this recipe out when your young ones aren't feeling so great.

Pear + Celery + Spinach

Fan Favorite!

Kids love this one, and so do parents! It's refreshingly simple, yet moving toward a more "green" centered juice. The celery is a fantastic base and will give the juice its volume. The spinach creates a beautiful and nutrient packed green color but is still mild enough for kids to accept it early on. The pear is the perfect companion to sweeten it up.

Pear + Apple + Spinach

Fan Favorite!

Adding pear to the popular and tasty Apple + Spinach combination sweetens the deal even more. This is a great recipe to use when starting out due to its sweet taste combined with the mild tasting green color.

"Eleven Alive"

Fan Favorite!

If you'd like to jump right into a big ingredient list, here's one for you that is already loved by kids. You can add pear to almost any green juice recipe to help sweeten it up for pickier taste buds. This juice has a bit of everything and is packed with energy and life!

1. Base veggies: **Celery + Cucumber**
2. Sweeteners: **Pear + Apple**
3. Greens: **Spinach + Kale**
4. Citrus: **Lemon + Lime**
5. Herbs and spices: **Cilantro + Parsley + Ginger**

Pineapple Juice

I have two words to describe this juice: liquid candy. It's best served in small chunks or in a smoothie because of the high sugar content. Water it down if you juice it, or try some coconut water for a tropical taste! You can also combine it with celery for a refreshing and delicious way to aid in hydration. If organic, just wash well and juice with skin. Otherwise, clean the skin well so that nothing is dragged into the fruit while cutting.

Nutrition:

Vitamins: A and C, B-complex vitamins, copper, manganese, and potassium.

Health Benefits:

- Tackles aches and pains after game day or sitting in class for long periods of time.
- Prevents and fights colds and cough.
- Aids in digestion.
- Strengthens bones.
- Helps to keep gums healthy.

Storage:

Keep a fresh pineapple on the counter or in the fridge for a couple of days, if you haven't eaten it already! Core and skin before freezing in an airtight container for up to 12 months.

Tip:

Pineapples stop ripening once they are harvested. When buying, opt for one with green and yellow colors, but no white. If the leaves look withered, move on to the next one.

Did You Know?

The pineapple got its name because it resembles a pine cone.

Use the top to grow a new pineapple at home. It'll take about 3 years!

Grape Juice

Imagine a grape juice that actually tastes like grapes instead of pure refined sugar! This is another fruit that should hit the stomach with its fiber along for the ride. A little note here: Unless you plan on peeling each one of them, grapes aren't really optimal for smoothies. But, grapes are a great way to change your picky eater's mind about juicing. Grape juice should be watered down with plain or coconut water to minimize the sugar intake, as well as to dilute the very sweet taste.

Nutrition:

Vitamins A, C and K, with micronutrient minerals like copper, iron, and manganese.

Health Benefits:

- Fights viral and fungal infections.
- Provides a natural anti-inflammatory.
- Relief for asthma, constipation, headaches, and fatigue.

Storage:

Keep grapes unwashed and in the refrigerator until ready to eat. You can also freeze them for a refreshing and tasty summer treat!

Tip:

Choose red grapes over white for their increased nutritional value.

Did You Know?

Grapes come in a variety of fun colors, including red, black, dark blue, yellow, green, orange, and pink. White grapes are actually considered to be green.

Watermelon Juice

As its name implies, the watermelon is made up of approximately 92% water. Watermelon juice isn't typically thought of as a "juice," however in some parts of the world it's not uncommon to see a pitcher of it right next to the orange juice at breakfast.

Nutrition:

Rich in Vitamins A, B1, B6 and C, manganese and potassium, antioxidants, lycopene.

Health Benefits:

Helps strengthen the immune system and aids in proper functioning of nerves, muscles, cardiovascular system and brain.

Storage:

Watermelon can be stored, uncut, at room temperature for about a week, and up to two weeks in the refrigerator.

Cut into small cubes and freeze for a sweet treat in the hot summer months.

Tips:

Try using watermelon juice to sweeten up plain water for a cool summer treat.

Juice watermelon, lemon, and coconut water for a refreshing sports drink alternative!

Peel the watermelon before juicing, and use taste preference as a guide to how much of the rind to remove. It can be bitter, but carries nutrients and is actually cooked and eaten on its own in China.

Did You Know?

The Japanese were the first to successfully grow square shaped watermelons which can be more easily stored inside of a fridge.

Tomato Juice

This vegetable juice is popular around the world. While it is often paired with other vegetables, it's also great to drink alone and kids love it! While drinking raw tomato juice, add a few drops of oil to aid in absorption of the fat-soluble lycopene.

Nutrition:

Rich in Vitamins A and C, B-complex vitamins, potassium, iron, calcium, and manganese.

Health Benefits:

- Helps fight fatigue.
- Boosts the immune system.
- Helps to protect the skin against sunburn.

Storage:

Tomatoes should be kept at room temperature to preserve flavor, and out of direct sunlight.

Tip:

Remove all greens and stem before juicing as they can be toxic. The fruit itself can be harmful to dogs if large amounts are consumed.

Did You Know?

There is a less common variety of tomato that has stripes and is called
"Green Zebra."

Tomato + Spinach

In addition to the benefits of tomatoes and spinach on their own, this combination also helps to relieve and prevent constipation. Start with one tomato and a handful of spinach. This juice is a perfect green juice starter for the tomato lover in your family.

"Better than a Salad"
Tomato + Cucumber + Red Bell Pepper + Lemon + Scallion + Parsley

This is a favorite amongst our clients! The red bell pepper adds a sweet taste, while the lemon gives it a little kick for fun. Kids who might otherwise shy away from onions may find that that they can tolerate or even enjoy the milder tasting scallion. This recipe will help with cold and flu, due in part to the antiviral properties of the scallion's allicin.

"Original B-8 Juice"
Tomato + Cucumber + Celery + Green Bell Pepper + Parsley + Ginger

The tomato will take center stage in this recipe. The green bell pepper isn't quite as sweet as a ripened red one, so this combination will be preferred by kids whose tastes have changed in favor of a less sweetened juice.

"Veggie Splash"

Bring the garden to their glass with this delicious and nutritious veggie splash! Put in several of the sweet tasting carrots to start and it will help mask the stronger taste of the garlic and ginger. Green onion is another name for scallion.

There are so many benefits to this combination, each serving will help keep your kids strong and full of healthy energy.

1. Base veggies: **Celery + Tomato**
2. Sweeteners: **Carrot**
3. Veggies: **Green Pepper + Green Onion**
4. Greens: **Spinach**
5. Citrus: **Lemon**
6. Herbs and spices: **Parsley + Garlic + Ginger**

Cucumbers

Cucumbers are what I use as a base for many of my green juices. They are made up of 96% water, and when juiced, are actually more effective in treating and preventing dehydration than plain water!

This juice is bitter on its own, and while some people won't mind the taste in order to feel the effects of a glass of pure cucumber juice, kids probably won't add it to their list of favorites. Then again, maybe yours will!

Nutrition:

Vitamins A, C, and K, silica (in the peel), and potassium.

Health Benefits:

Silica helps keep connective tissue strong... important for holding the body together.

Silica is found in intracellular cement, muscles, tendons, ligaments, bone and cartilage.

Cucumber juice helps with skin complexion.

Storage:

Unless it's very hot and humid where you live, you can leave cucumbers at room temperature, but keep them away from tomatoes. If storing them in the fridge, wrap them loosely in a paper towel.

Tip:

To reduce the bitter taste of cucumber juice in recipes, remove the seeds. Add them back in gradually as your child's taste preference changes.

Did You Know?

Botanically speaking, cucumbers are accessory fruits. But, much like tomatoes, they are most often thought of as vegetables.

Cucumber + Apple

Simple combinations like this are perfect for convincing kids new to juicing that it tastes great. The cucumber gives it a watery base, which is perfect for hydration, and pairs beautifully with the apple for a sweet treat. Remember to remove the bitter seeds and peel of the cucumber for beginners, and add them back later for the additional nutrients.

"Capri Kiddie Juice"
Cucumber + Apple + Broccoli

Our juicing community members have been serving this juice to their kids with great success. What's not to love? Adding the broccoli is fun and helps fight the common cold by strengthening the immune system.

"Night Night Sleep Tight Juice"
Cucumber + Bok Choy + Lemon + Spinach

Make this juice for the little insomniac in your house. The calcium in dark leafy greens such as bok choy and spinach will help slow them down in a safe and natural way. The magnesium in the spinach will help the body absorb the calcium. Nighty-night!

"My Memory, Oh My!"

To help with studying and exam days, juice up your kids with this memory enhancing recipe. Peppermint helps to increase alertness and memory in a much safer way than the popular canned choices. The base vegetables will help keep them hydrated which will keep their concentration and brain function in check.

1. Base veggies: **Cucumber + Celery**
2. Sweeteners: **Carrot + Apple**
3. Citrus: **Lemon**
4. Herbs and spices: **Parsley + Ginger + Mint to jazz it up!**

Celery

This one might be unusual as a stand-alone juice, but some find that they like the unique flavor. It's also one of the best bases to start out with when acclimating tummies of the young, and not-so-young, to juicing. It is one of the easiest of the greens to digest and tolerate, along with cucumbers and fennel.

Nutrition:

Vitamins A, C, and K, folic acid, riboflavin, niacin, sodium, potassium, calcium, manganese and magnesium.

Health Benefits:

- Use as a diuretic.
- Great for an after workout or after the game drink.
- Contains coumarins which help with migraines.
- Helps boost the immune system.

Storage:

Celery will keep fresh longer if sealed in a plastic bag in the fridge. You can also wrap it in foil and it will stay fresh for a few weeks... but who's going to have celery in the fridge for that long when there is a juicer on the counter?

Tip:

Buy from the organic section, and wash the ribs thoroughly. Fresh celery will snap, not bend.

Did You Know?

Celery is part of the carrot, parsley, and fennel family. Celery juice has a "cooling" effect when you drink it.

Celery + Apple

A great way to introduce celery juice is to pair it with the sweet apple taste that kids already love. Start with red apples and switch to green once their taste buds stop craving sugary juices. Jazz up simple juices like this one with a knuckle of ginger.

Celery + Carrot + Apple

Use a couple of stalks of celery, a couple of carrots, and one green apple for a refreshing and sweet juice that is kid-approved. One step further than celery and apple together, introducing carrots will "up" the juicing game.

"Muscle Cramp Stopper"
Celery + Carrot + Asparagus

Cramps can sometimes be caused by dehydration, so juicing with a watery base such as celery or cucumber is a good start. Asparagus is also high in Vitamins C & E which help to combat muscle cramps. The asparagus has a stronger flavor, so use the sweetness of the carrots to help this combination go down smoothly.

Celery + Cucumber + Carrot + Lemon

Simple, mild, sweet, with a bit of zing... already loved by many kids and sure to be a new favorite of many more! This is the perfect recipe for introducing both celery and lemon. A couple of stalks of celery and ¼ of a lemon are perfect for beginners.

"Bone Builder"
Celery + Carrot + Parsley + Lemon

The celery, with its benefits toward bone health, is what names this combination. Use several stalks of celery, a few carrots, about ¼ cup of parsley, and ¼ - ½ lemon, depending on preference. Don't forget the green juice mustache!

"The Celery Cooler"
Celery + Cucumber + Tomato + Cilantro

Perfect for those hot summer nights, this combination will cool them down after playing outside all day. Celery has a calming effect on the nervous system and will help regulate body temperature. First juice the tomato, then the cucumber, celery, and cilantro.

"Detoxifying Celery Juice"
Celery + Apple + Carrot + Beet + Parsley

With three sources of sweetness in this recipe, it's perfect for serving to young ones who need to clean out their systems, or "detox." Start with the celery as a base and use 3 carrots, 1 apple, and ½ of a beet with green roots to sweeten it up. One cup of parsley may seem like a lot, but the cleansing effects are well worth it.

Beet

Whether or not you liked the taste of cooked beets as a kid, juicing the beet with other flavors helps mask the earthy taste that kids might not like. Juice beets sparingly with young children, since drinking too much can cause an overload of minerals in the liver.

Nutrition:

Vitamins A and C (mostly in the greens), B-complex vitamins, folate, iron, manganese, copper, and magnesium.

Health Benefits:

- Is a powerful antioxidant that builds the body's immunity.
- May prevent anemia.
- Enhances athletic performance.

Storage:

Remove stems before storing in the refrigerator. If kept in a bag in the crisper, beet bulbs can stay fresh for 1-2 weeks.

Tips:

* The red beet is sweeter than yellow, and yellow's flavor is earthier than the others.
* Consuming too many beets could cause urine to turn a pink color. Use caution when adding as a regular part of your child's diet.
* Start with only about ¼ of a small beet per serving for young children.

Did You Know?

* Beet pulp is sometimes used in place of hay for horses that may be allergic, and also fed to horses that are in training.
* Beets have been used medicinally for relief from headaches and toothaches.

Cucumber + Apple + Beet

Fan favorite!

This is a fun, colorful, and tasty way to introduce juiced beets! The cucumber gives it volume and hydrates, while both the apple and beet sweeten the deal. Use red beets to give this juice its gorgeous color and taste that kids will love.

"Energizer Bunny"
Beet + Spinach + Broccoli + Lemon

Get your little bunny hopping to the—wait for it—"beet" with this fun and nutritious juice that is packed with energy! Spinach and other dark leafy greens contain folate which may help decrease the risk of depression. Beets are high in healthy carbohydrates which fuel the body in a nutritious way.

Apple + Carrot + Beet + Kale

Fan favorite!

FitLife kids have given this recipe a big thumbs up! How could they resist drinking a glass of kale juice with all of this nutritious sweetness dancing on the tongue? Reduce the amount of apple and carrot as your young ones get used to the taste of kale.

Carrot + Beet + Spinach + Lemon + Ginger

Fan favorite!

Turn up the sweet with carrots and beet! Spinach has a milder taste compared to other dark leafy greens, so it's perfect for a starter green juice. Use two or three carrots, half of a beet, a handful of spinach, ¼ - ½ lemon with peel if organic, and about ½ inch of ginger. Yum!

"Ginger Lemon Blast"

Fan favorite!

A classic combination of nutrient dense and flavor-packed juices, this particular mix will leave your taste buds and your little ones begging for more. This is one of our favorites at FitLife and is one of our go-to juices when we have guests in town. You can't go wrong with the Ginger Lemon Blast.

1. Base veggies: Cucumber + Celery
2. Sweeteners: Apple + Beet
3. Greens: Kale
4. Citrus: Lemon
5. Herbs and spices: Ginger

"Beetastic"

Fan favorite!

If you were looking for a great way to introduce ginger, this is it. The sweet flavors of apple, carrot, and beet will help mask the more intense ones of ginger and spinach. Juice up those little bodies with this powerhouse of nutrition and taste!

1. Base veggies: **Cucumber + Celery**
2. Sweeteners: **Apple + Carrot + Beet**
3. Greens: **Spinach**
4. Citrus: **Lemon**
5. Herbs and spices: **Ginger**

Lemon

Lemons are most commonly consumed as a juice and has been loved for generations as the refreshing summer drink mixed with sugar and ice: lemonade. It has also inspired many young entrepreneurs to learn the basics of business. What's not to love about that? Add ¼ to ½ of a small lemon to almost any juice recipe to give it a little kick.

Nutrition:

Rich in Vitamin C, B-complex vitamins, and a small amount of Vitamin A. Lemons also provide minerals such as iron, copper, calcium and potassium.

Health Benefits:

- Aids in digestion.
- Acts as an antibacterial force inside the stomach.
- Cleans the liver and flushes toxins from the body.

Storage:

Store lemons in a sealed plastic bag and in the refrigerator; they will last a few weeks.

Tip:

To prepare a lemon for juicing, first remove the peel. If it's organic, you can leave it on, but know that the peel will have a bitter taste that other ingredients in the recipe may not be able to mask.

Did You Know?

* There are nearly a dozen different varieties of lemon. One of them is pink! The variety most commonly found in supermarkets is called "Eureka."
* If you attach electrodes to lemons, it will produce enough electricity to power a light bulb. Try it out for a fun at-home science experiment!

"Fresh Lemonade / Limeade"
Apple + Lemon / + Lime

Granulated sugar need not apply. Juicing two apples per lemon, with a dilution rate of 1:1, gives you the perfect refresher for a sunny summer day. Add lime for a variation on this timeless favorite.

Lemon + Apple + Carrot + Spinach

Fan favorite!

Trees meet garden in this easy to digest fruit and vegetable combination. It has the perfect blend of sweet and tart. The spinach adds the unmistakable taste of dark leafy greens but in a mild way, so kids will love it.

"Go-Go Juice"
Cucumber + Celery + Apple + Lemon + Ginger

Busy day ahead? Parents need a lot of energy to keep up with the youngest members of the family. Don't let your get-up-and-go go without you. Share this energy packed juice recipe in the morning, and get ready for a day full of productivity and action!

Cucumber + Celery + Apple + Spinach + Lemon + Cilantro

Cilantro gives a kick to but also blends into this tried and true combination. It is a natural and powerful detoxifier as well, helping to remove heavy metals from body tissue. Wrap the cilantro in the spinach to extract the most juice from its tiny leaves.

"Green Lemonade"

Let's get serious about our lemonade, shall we? Keep the apple and lemon in the spotlight, but kick up the nutrients a few notches with some green and let the ginger finish it off with a kick of spice. This isn't your grandmother's lemonade! We're confident that it'll quickly become a new favorite for your kids to pass on to their kids.

1. Base veggies: **Celery**
2. Sweeteners: **Apple**
3. Greens: **Romaine Lettuce + Kale**
4. Citrus: **Lemon**
5. Herbs & spices: **Ginger**

Kale

"Kale" is one of the newest buzzwords when talking about health foods. Yes, it's a dark leafy green, so it will have a bitter taste to the untrained taste bud. It's also super packed with what your kids need to grow strong. Kale is used in a many of the juice recipes we love most. Check out the FitLife Kids Menu for some irresistible kale treat recipes!

Nutrition:

Vitamins A and C, beta carotene, calcium, potassium.

Health Benefits:

- Is a fantastic anti-inflammatory.
- Builds the body's immune system.
- Helps keep skin healthy.
- The chlorophyll in kale helps with bad breath.

Storage:

Store in a plastic bag in the refrigerator for up to a week. Do not wash until ready to use.

Tips:

Although all have a stronger green leaf taste, Lacinato kale is slightly sweeter than its curly cousin, and red kale is the sweetest of the three.

One or two kale leaves added to a recipe is enough for one juice serving.

Kale is high in calcium, so be sure to get enough Vitamin D to aid in absorption.

Did You Know?

Lacinato Kale is sometimes called Dinosaur Kale. See how many different green juices you and your kids can assign dinosaur names to!

Apple + Carrot + Kale

Fan favorite!

Graduating from the milder spinach to the stronger taste of kale is easy with this simple recipe. Packed with nutrients and sweetness, you could call this one Sweet Stegosaurus Juice. Kids have already given a thumbs up to the taste, and a cool dinosaur name adds the fun!

Cucumber + Celery + Apple + Kale

Trade in the sweetness of the previous recipe for volume with this one's water packed cucumber and celery. The apple is still enough to keep it sweet, but with a deliberate move toward a greener juice.

Cucumber + Apple + Kale + Lemon + Ginger

Add a little sass to the trio of cucumber, apple, and kale with about ¼ of a lemon and ¼ - ½ inch of ginger. When your family is ready to give up the sweeter taste of apples in red, switch it up for a green one to create one of the healthiest and easiest combinations that kids love.

Cucumber + Celery + Apple + Kale + Lime + Ginger

Celery will team up with the cucumber to give more base volume to this juice. Limes are fun to add because, though they are related to lemons, they bring their own unique flavor to to the mix. They tend to be a bit sweeter, and bring a higher concentration of Vitamin C, as well.

Nutritionally superb and friendly to little taste buds, this recipe is a sure winner for the whole family to enjoy.

"The Green Trampoline"

This juice will get those juveniles jumpin' in no time flat, or... about ten minutes. Promote hydration with about ½ of the cucumber as a base for a kid-sized serving, and add one green apple to sweeten it up. Use one leaf each of the greens, and ½ of a lemon to bring it to the next level. Switch the lemon out for lime for an all-green version of this juice. Feeling a bit run-down? Prepare an extra serving for yourself!

1. Base veggie: **Cucumber**
2. Sweetener: **Apple**, preferably a green one
3. Greens: **Cabbage + Chard + Collard Greens + Romaine + Kale**
4. Citrus: **Lemon**

Spinach

Not just for cartoon sailors anymore, spinach is actually loved by many kids all over the world! It's a dark leafy green, but has a milder flavor. It's perfect for adding to green juices for young ones, as well as adults, who are a little nervous about drinking the color green. Add a handful to any juice to pack in the nutrition and make your kids feel like they can save the world.

Nutrition:

Rich in iron, Vitamins A, C, and K, B-complex vitamins, copper, magnesium, manganese, potassium, selenium, and zinc.

Health Benefits:

- Fantastic as an anti-inflammatory and infection fighter.
- Promotes healthy skin.
- Helps promote a healthy nervous system and brain function.

Storage:

Spinach should be dry when stored, so do not wash it first. Place in a paper bag, loosely wrapped in a paper towel, and keep refrigerated for up to a week.

Tips:

* Spinach is on the list of most heavily pesticide-contaminated, so choose organic.
* As with most greens, use spinach each day for only up to 4 days, and then switch to a different green leafy veggie.

Did You Know?

China is the world leader in production of spinach, followed by the United States.

In medieval times, artists would use spinach juice as pigment for green ink or paint.

Apple + Carrot + Spinach

Fan favorite

You really can't go wrong with this trifecta of awesomeness. Not only does this have an amazing impact on your palate, it is easy to consume and is loaded with vitamins and phytonutrients. For an additional treat, mix in some homemade almond milk. The fat from the almonds acts like a transport, helping the body to absorb more of the Vitamin A in the carrots. Enjoy!

"Sleep Better Sally"
Celery + Spinach + Kale + Lemon

Do your young ones often feel restless and have trouble falling asleep? Let this recipe help them rest easy tonight. I personally love this combination because the kale is loaded with magnesium which promotes better sleep safely and naturally. Sleep tight!

"Recharge Your Alkaline Battery"
Cucumber + Cabbage + Spinach + Lemon

As I sat one day with Jay Kordich, a mentor and personal friend, he shared with me that one of his favorite foods to juice is red cabbage. It has an amazing flavor and is loaded with Vitamin U, which has been proven to help heal ulcers. This recipe will also help relieve bloating and excess gas, which often cause tummy aches.

"Energizing Power Drink"
Carrot + Spinach + Parsley + Ginger

Step away from that store-bought energy drink. This juice recipe will not only give you the energy you need, but will give your body the power it needs to help you not just get through the day, but conquer it. Teens especially love the quick fix of a high energy formula, and this one will deliver long after consumed.

Celery + Apple + Carrot + Kale + Spinach

FitLife families love this recipe. The ingredients are easy to find, it's easy to juice them up, and the amazing taste makes it really easy to drink! This power-packed combo is perfect for those rushed moments when you need a delicious burst of immediate energy.

"Iron Man Juice"

The Iron Man Juice is the perfect recipe if you're looking to add some iron to your little one's juice without them noticing. Spinach and romaine are loaded with iron, a nutrient that is needed to make hemoglobin, which carries oxygen to the body's cells.

1. Base veggies: **Cucumber + Celery**
2. Sweeteners: **Apple + Carrot**
3. Greens: **Spinach + Romaine**
4. Herbs and spices: **Parsley**

Parsley

Parsley is certainly a nice way to fancy up a plate at mealtime, but juicing it is more nutritious! The leaves are small, but they're packed with flavor and healthy goodness. If you're unsure about introducing parsley to a picky young eater, try hiding it in juice recipes that already contain a leafy green or two.

Nutrition:

Antioxidants, Vitamins A, C and K, folate, iron, calcium, magnesium, potassium, copper, and manganese, chlorophyll, beta carotene.

Health Benefits:

- Anti-inflammatory and potent detoxifier.
- Boosts the immune system.
- Good for upset tummies because it stimulates digestive enzymes.
- Helps raise energy levels for long days at school or before physical activities.
- Has been shown to raise glutathione levels. Read more at altmedicine.about.com.

Storage:

Trim the ends of the stems and place leaf side up in a glass with a small amount of water. Loosely cover the top with plastic and refrigerate for up to a week.

Tips:

* Some people believe that flat-leafed, or Italian, parsley has a stronger flavor.
* Wrap parsley inside larger leafy greens to help squeeze out the most juice.

Did You Know?

Another type of parsley is grown as a root vegetable commonly used in central and eastern parts of Europe in soups or stews, but also eaten raw like a carrot.

"L.A. Lung Juice"
Celery + Parsley + Watercress

The great thing about this combination is that the celery hides the more intense flavors of the parsley and watercress.

If you read my first book ⬚u⬚in⬚⬚é⬚⬚es ⬚or ⬚ ita⬚it⬚ an⬚ ⬚ ed⬚⬚, you'll see that the amazing watercress also makes an appearance in a few of the recipes there.

This juice is perfect for people wanting to detox their lungs and may also help clear up congestion.

"Super Human Super Powers"

Any time you can include cilantro, parsley, and ginger in the same recipe and it tastes absolutely amazing, you have a winning combination. That's what you get with the Super Human Super Powers juice. It's named for its ability to leave your immune system giving you a standing ovation.

1. Sweeteners: **Apple + Carrot**
2. Citrus: **Lemon**
3. Herbs and spices: **Parsley + Cilantro + Ginger + Garlic**

"The Great Explorer"

Fan favorite!

If your children imagine themselves climbing the highest mountains and diving to the depths of the ocean, tell them that all great explorers should drink this before leaving home for their next journey beyond the driveway. It's a great juice for energy production, and is an excellent way to prepare them for big adventures in the backyard or on the soccer field.

1. Base veggies: **Cucumber + Celery**
2. Sweeteners: **Apple + Carrot**
3. Greens: **Kale + Spinach**
4. Citrus: **Lemon**
5. Herbs and spices: **Parsley**

Ginger

This spice has everything nice! Use ginger to give any recipe a little kick. When I add it to juice recipes I use a large amount, but I'm also the guy who will chew on it raw and love it! When starting out, use a small piece... about ¼ of an inch sliced. See how they like it, and let me know if I have any fellow young ginger lovers out there!

Nutrition:

Vitamins B6, C & E, calcium, iron, magnesium, manganese, potassium, selenium.

Health Benefits:

- Ginger is a powerful anti-inflammatory and pain reducer..
- Often used as a remedy for motion sickness and relieves nausea.
- Antiviral to help heal and prevent colds and flu.
- Boiled in water and used as a tea, ginger can help soothe sore throats.

Storage:

Place unwashed fresh ginger root in a sealed plastic bag and refrigerate for 2-3 weeks.

Tips:

Some people may be sensitive to ginger and experience what is called the "ginger jitters" if they consume too much of it. Keep the amounts low for children, and check with your child's pediatrician if you have any concerns.

When buying, look for a piece with the least amount of branching.

Did You Know?

Ginger root is actually not a root at all, but a "rhizome," and individual branches of the rhizome are known as "hands."

"Mighty Mouse Juice Recipe"
Apple + Ginger

Your kids will feel like they're wearing a cape after enjoying this simple and delicious recipe for cold prevention. Use two apples and about ¼ inch slice of ginger to start. Increase the amount of ginger as their little buds get accustomed to the taste.

"Vitamin Booster: Cold & Flu"
Apple + Carrot + Ginger

The FitLife team is blessed to have a Naturopathic doctor on speed dial to give us the inside scoop on how to heal and keep the body strong. What we've learned is that oftentimes a cold will start in the gut, and this is why we love to add ginger to many of our juice recipes. Ginger is a ninja when it comes to boosting the immune system and helping your young ones combat colds and flu.

"Anti-inflammatory Juice"
Carrot + Cabbage + Parsley + Ginger

This recipe will be well accepted by children whose taste buds have gotten used to juicing vegetables without the added sweetness of fruits. The ginger is pungent, aromatic, and oftentimes very spicy (depending on how much is used).

Generations have used ginger for the benefits of its potent anti-inflammatory compounds called gingerols. These are believed to help reduce pain levels and increase mobility for people with osteoarthritis or rheumatoid arthritis. An anti-inflammatory remedy is also a must-have for all active kids.

"Princess Jasmine's Fav"
Cucumber + Carrot + Lemon + Watercress + Ginger

Help raise the drawbridge and keep colds out of the castle with this delicious recipe for cold prevention. It also helps young princes and princesses shake off nausea so that they can have an enchanted time at the royal ball. Kings and queens will love this combination for its overall nutritional quality. FitLife approved for royal families everywhere.

Garlic

Legendary for its ability to protect against scary long-toothed night people and the slightly less menacing mosquito, garlic packs a punch when it comes to keeping us healthy. It's a fairly potent addition to our food, so you might be wondering how much stronger it'll be when juiced! I wouldn't recommend juicing it alone, but it's a fantastic addition to vegetable juices. We've included a few recipes that have already been tested and loved by kids.

Nutrition:

Garlic is rich in calcium, iron, magnesium, manganese, potassium, selenium, zinc, and is high in Vitamins A, B6 and C.

Health Benefits:

- Has antiviral, antibacterial, and antifungal properties.
- Used in Chinese medicine to treat cold, cough, and bronchitis.
- Boosts the immune system.

Storage:

Store whole store-bought garlic bulbs in a dry, dark place for several months. Once peeled, store cloves in a clear plastic container and refrigerate for up to three weeks.

Tip:

Wrap the garlic in parsley leaves while juicing to prevent garlic breath.

Did You Know?

* Leaves and flowers of the garlic plant are edible, with a milder flavor than the bulb.
* Garlic flowers do not produce seeds. New plants are created by planting the cloves.
* Due to its overpowering taste and smell, it has been nicknamed the "stinking rose."
* Celebrate National Garlic Day on April 19th every year!

Apple + Carrot + Lemon + Ginger + Garlic

With any sign of a cold coming on, this is one of the first juice combinations I'll reach for. Use just enough apple and carrot to give it a mildly sweet taste, and let the lemon, ginger, and garlic take care of the rest. FitLifers agree that this is a great recipe to offer anyone who is curious about the juice that you're drinking.

"Infection and Virus Fighter"
Apple + Carrot + Beet + Lemon + Garlic

We know that you would rather head to the kitchen for nature's antibiotic before walking into a pharmacy. This is a simple and delicious juice that many have settled on as their first choice when illness takes hold. Your young ones will love the sweet combination of flavors as the garlic works hard to help them feel better fast.

"A Kicking Juice"

If the taste of garlic isn't on your list of favorites but you want the health benefits it brings, you'll want to try this recipe. Start with one clove of garlic and give it a taste test. We think that the garlic and ginger combo is amazing, and you'll love the alkalizing effects of the lemon. If you're looking for a juice that will kick your energy up, this should do the trick.

1. Base veggie: **Cucumber**
2. Sweeteners: **Carrot + Apple + Beet**
3. Citrus: **Lemon**
4. Herbs and spices: **Garlic + Ginger**

Wheatgrass

Bring the juice bar home to your kitchen! A little goes a long way in helping to restore and maintain optimal health. Wheatgrass is one of the most nutritious foods on the planet. We love it, and your kids will be surprised that grass can actually taste sweet!

Nutrition:

Packed with Vitamins A, B, C, and E. Contains calcium, iron, magnesium, potassium, essential amino acids, and is a rockstar source of chlorophyll.

Health Benefits:

* Aids in digestion.
* Is a powerful detoxifier.
* Increases blood flow, which boosts energy levels and promotes faster metabolism.
* Helps clear up acne and improve the appearance of scars.
* Soothes sore throats when gargled.

Storage:

Juice harvested wheatgrass immediately. Store uncut bunches unwashed for up to a week in the refrigerator.

Tip:

Adults should consume no more than 4 ounces per day. Serve only 1-2 ounces to children, as it can cause upset stomach in higher amounts.

Did You Know?

* Wheatgrass does not contain gluten. Gluten is part of the wheat grain.

* You can grow and harvest wheatgrass very easily at home! This would make a fun project for the whole family.

Cucumber + Apple + Carrot + Wheatgrass + Mint

This recipe is a smart choice; the early Romans believed that eating mint would increase their intelligence. It improves concentration, too! Teens will want to try a little of the mint juice topically to treat blackheads on the surface of the skin.

"Sweet & Sassy Grass"

The name serves this juice combination well, with its splash of sweetness and sassy kick of the garlic and ginger. This juice packs a powerful nutritional punch and is loaded with antioxidants that will keep your body going until the day is done. Bear in mind that garlic is extremely potent in small doses; one clove is enough to start with.

1. Sweeteners: **Apple + Carrot + Beet**
2. Greens: **Kale + Wheatgrass**
3. Herbs and spices: **Garlic + Ginger**

Green Juice Builder #1

Carrot + Cucumber

Many kids will like the sweet taste of carrot juice alone, so it's a great one to start with while introducing more vegetables. Start with one or two carrots, and add green by including half of a cucumber with the bitter seeds and peel removed. Together they form a taste that is mild and sweet. Over time and as those young taste buds grow accustomed to drinking less sweetened juices, you can add the peel and seeds back in.

Carrot + Cucumber, next add Apple

If the carrot and cucumber pairing is still being met with upturned noses, try adding half of an apple to sweeten it up, or a whole one if that's what they prefer. You can reduce the amount of apple over time as they get used to drinking their vegetables. This combination is a Juicing Vegetables fan favorite!

Carrot + Cucumber + Apple, next add Spinach

This next step really brings in the green, but in a mild way. Spinach is packed with nutrients, but doesn't have the bitter taste of many of the dark leafy greens. A handful of spinach is plenty. This will go a long way to show kids that green can still be delicious.

Carrot + Cucumber + Apple + Spinach, next add Kale

Start with only one kale leaf at first, and add more when the taste buds start to beg for it. The idea of the juice builders is to gradually build up from a single juice, such as the carrot juice we started with for this builder, and end with 5 ingredients for a delicious and nutritious green juice that is still mild enough for beginners and kids to love.

Green Juice Builder #2

Pear + Celery

Pear juice is very sweet on its own, but adding celery as a watery base makes a beautiful light green and delicious way to introduce a vegetable to a juice glass. Pear juice should be watered down anyway, due to its high sugar content. Celery is the perfect way to do it!

Start with one pear and a few stalks of celery. You can also challenge your child to switch the celery with cucumber for a taste test, which will show them that recipes can always be altered based on what they like.

Pear + Celery, next add Red Bell Pepper

Many people don't even think of bell peppers for juicing, but they make a great addition. Green peppers have a bitter taste, but the red ones are sweet and work well to include in a mild juice. You don't need a lot, unless you want the taste be dominant. Start with ¼ of a small one.

Pear + Celery + Red Bell Pepper, next add Broccoli

Now for the little "trees." This will turn the juice a beautiful darker green. We've included broccoli to help you think outside the box when it comes to juicing. If it has water content, juice it! You and your child can make up a fun name for this combination, such as Sweet Forest.

Pear + Celery + Red Bell Pepper + Broccoli, next add Romaine Lettuce

Romaine leaves aren't quite as bitter as kale, featured in the first juice builder, so this one will stay on the mild side. It's great for getting the little ones thinking about putting green leaves into the juicer and have the result still be delicious and kid approved. You can try adding a little kick to each of these juice builder combinations by including ¼ of a small lemon.

Green Juice Builder #3

Pear + Cucumber

As mentioned in Builder #2, you can switch the celery with cucumber as a partner to pear juice. It's sweet and refreshing! Try one pear with ½ of a cucumber. For this juice builder, you can also substitute celery for each progression and it'll still taste great. You can also replace the pear with apple. Have fun experimenting to find what your kids like best!

Pear + Cucumber, next add Bok Choy

Not only is it fun to say, but Bok Choy is a great addition to juicing! It has a high water content and mild taste to go along with the low calories and nutritional benefits. Start with one leaf and add more as desired.

Pear + Cucumber + Bok Choy, next add Green Leaf Lettuce

Green Leaf Lettuce is another addition that will convince young taste buds that green can taste great. A few leaves will do it. You could exchange it for red leaf lettuce, as well. This is a delicious salad in a glass. :)

Pear + Cucumber + Bok Choy + Green Leaf Lettuce, next add Kale

And back to one of my favorites: Kale. Just a leaf of this will turn this juice builder into a nutrition packed but mild-tasting juice that is sure to please. Kale is added in the last step because it does have a bitter taste. When added to the other ingredients, the bitter is masked, but the amazing nutritional qualities of the juice take center stage.

Top 5 Juicing Add-Ons

Add some pizzazz to your family's favorite juice recipes with these popular add-ons! They give any juice an additional blast of nutrition without compromising on great taste. In fact, we think they taste amazing! Mix and match with almost any juice recipe.

Coconut Oil

It's one of the most bioavailable fats on the planet, and we love adding it to nearly everything! Hair, skin, juices, and food... there really are no limits. Your kids will absolutely love its amazing flavor, and you'll love its benefits which include strengthening the immune system, its antifungal and antibacterial properties, and that it improves digestion and nutrient absorption.

Apple Cider Vinegar

What is not to love about ACV? I often add 2 tablespoons to my morning juice to clear up toxins and give me massive amounts of solid energy. Medical research shows that it offers amazing health benefits such as helping with acne, allergies, flu, heartburn, chronic fatigue syndrome, and sore throat.

Pink Salt

Most people, including your kiddos, are deficient in minerals. Pink salt is a super easy way to get many of the minerals the body needs. Just a dash of pink salt in their juice will increase their energy, restore health, aid in absorption of other nutrients, and enhance the overall flavor of the recipe.

Turmeric Powder

Dazzle your kids with the bright color and vibrant taste of this incredible root. Their little taste buds will thank you! Add either fresh raw turmeric or powder to their juice for a sweet and tangy taste they'll love. Turmeric is liken to gold in my house.

Oregano Oil

Is your little one feeling a little blue with maybe a stomachache or perhaps the flu? Help their little bodies fight these symptoms with a natural approach. Oregano is a natural antibiotic and has been shown to eliminate the bad kind of bacteria that can cause harm to your youngster's health. It doesn't take much; just a few drops of this oil in their juice will get them back on their feet.

Smoothies

As much as I love juicing, making green smoothies is another one of my favorites... and kids love them, too! Smoothies are a great way to consume your fruits, since you are actually blending them with the fiber intact. The fiber in fruits is needed to aid in digestion, which is the reason why they should be eaten whole or blended as a smoothie, as opposed to juicing them.

It's also important to chew your smoothies before swallowing. It may sound strange, but there's a very good reason for it. Digestion actually begins in the mouth, and chewing is part of the process of complete digestion.

The same rule for juicing applies to smoothies: Try to keep the fruits and vegetables separate or the fruits to a minimum while transitioning to greens. The exception would be for a green smoothie in which you can add an apple or pear.

Leafy vegetables are a great source of protein, chlorophyll, oxygen and phytonutrients. Blending them into a delicious drink is a great way to pack young bodies with the "right stuff" without them having to munch on a great big salad to get the same effect.

Recipes

Orange + Grapefruit + Lemon

For the citrus lovers in your family, this is a delicious way to pack in the Vitamin C and antioxidants for a powerful boost in the morning. Try starting out with one orange, ½ of a grapefruit, ¼ of a lemon. As with most recipes, let taste be your guide for determining amounts of each ingredient.

Orange + Banana + Avocado + Spinach

Go green with this delicious and simple recipe that is kid-approved. Loaded with potassium, this smoothie will help relieve anxiety and stress and enhances higher brain function such as learning and memory. Homework will be a snap! They'll feel great after enjoying this combination of sweet and rich flavors!

Apple + Carrot + Banana + Pineapple

This amazing blend of great tasting fruits welcomes the sweet tasting carrot for a delicious combination that your kids will love. Take it outside with you for a walk in the park or include it on the menu for your next camping trip with the family for a perfect summer afternoon treat. Add coconut oil for a tropical taste.

Strawberries + Blueberries + Spinach

Great for an energy boost, this is a recipe that your kids will ask for again and again. Blueberries have a lower sugar content than most other fruits and are loaded with healthy fats that are good for brain health. With these sweet flavors, they'll barely notice that there's spinach along for the ride. Add homemade almond milk for a smoother texture.

Celery + Apple + Banana + Kale + Lime

Call it a shake. Call it a smoothie. You could even call it a vegan ice cream. So delicious! Already approved by next generation FitLifers, we're sure your kids will love it, too. Add crushed ice and emerge from the kitchen with this cool treat to impress your guests who are visiting on a weekend afternoon.

Healthy Mint-Chocolate Chip Shake

Drive right through the drive-thru without stopping and hurry home to make some sweet shake magic in your own blender. When I sit down to describe the taste of this combination, all I can say is "I love." So will your kids. Hint: You, too, can indulge your senses with none of the guilt!

1. 1 frozen large banana, as ripe as possible
2. handful of cacao nibs
3. handful of mint
4. 2/3 cup coconut milk
5. frozen spinach (1/4 cup)
6. Blend everything together in your Vitamix or blender and enjoy.

PART THREE:

RECIPES FROM THE FITLIFE KITCHEN

FITLIFE APPROVED GROCERY LIST

Fitlife.tv Approved Kid Eats

Breakfast

* Captain Carrot Kids Juice
* Chia Seed Chocolate Smoothie
* Almond Butter & Banana Pancakes
* Green Smoothie

Lunch

* Mini Frittata Muffins
* Sun Dried Tomato Meatballs with Creamy Pesto
* Super Celery Juice

Dinner

* The New Lean "Happier Meal" Chicken Nuggets
* Not Your Normal Nachos

Snacks

* Guacamole Eggs
* Jicama Chips & Guacamole Dip
* Sweet Potato Rounds

Treats

* "Cheesy" Fitlife Popcorn
* Dairy Free Tapioca Pudding
* Surprise Kale Two Ways

Captain Carrot Kids Juice

Carrots are an amazing source of beta-carotene and are loaded with essential vitamins. The high amounts of vitamin A found in carrots benefit everything from vision to skin, and contain anti-aging properties. Kids love the natural sweet flavor of carrots and will have sustainable, healthy energy with which to start their day!

- 1 cucumber
- ½ golden beet
- 2 carrots
- 1 apple

Chia Seed Chocolate Smoothie

Chia seeds are an amazing superfood that boasts gut-healing properties and contains omega-3 fatty acids that are critical for brain function. Optimize your children's digestion and brainpower today!

- ½ cup Full fat coconut milk (Thai kitchen-canned is the best)
- 1 scoop chocolate protein powder
- ½ cup strawberries
- ½ frozen banana

- 1 tbsp. cocoa powder
- 1 tbsp chia seeds
- 1 large handful fresh spinach
- Option: add 2 tsp cinnamon to taste. This is a great way to moderate blood sugar levels, helping to prevent big blood sugar spikes from sweeter item such as banana and strawberries. Also, add ice for texture/volume.

Directions:

Mix chia seeds and coconut milk – let seeds expand for at least 15mins. Combine all ingredients in a VitaMix or blender. Add water or coconut milk (canned or carton-kind) if needed.

Almond Butter & Banana Pancakes

These pancakes will have the kids asking for seconds! They are healthful and easy to create. The almond butter and bananas create an amazing flavor. Bananas help soothe the tummy by strengthening the stomach lining and protecting against stomach acid. The potassium found in bananas is essential to countless cell functions and blood pressure.

- 2 ripe bananas
- 1 egg
- 1 heaping tablespoon of almond butter

Directions:

Mix bananas, eggs, and almond butter in a bowl.

- Stir in almond butter.
- Heat coconut oil or butter in a pan.
- Pour pancake mix into pan, flip, plate.

- Serve with blackberries or alternate berry of choice.

Green Smoothie

Almond milk and coconut milk offer a wonderful alternative to dairy products and kids love the creamy flavor of both. This recipe offers a great vehicle for amazing foods like kale, blueberries, and some extra protein with a protein powder.

- 1 cup Almond milk (nut milk) or coconut milk (unsweetened if possible)
- 3-5 leaves of kale
- ½ blueberries (or blackberries/strawberries, etc.)
- 1-2 scoops vanilla protein powder of your choice

Directions:

- In a VitaMix or blender, mix all ingredients.
- Option to add ice for texture and/or volume.

Mini Frittata Muffins

This recipe works wonders for school lunches, and is a super easy pack-and-go snack option. Eliminate excuses for low quality quick meals when it comes to your kids – make some muffins ahead of time and be prepared for days! Yields 12.

- 15 eggs (Use 15 in silicone muffin pans, use 12 eggs for metal muffin tins or individual silicone cups.)
- 1-2 tsp. pepper
- 1-2 tsp. sea salt

- 2 cups various chopped veggies such as blanched broccoli, red pepper, zucchini, mushrooms, etc.
- ½ cup onion diced small
- Optional: ½ - 1 cup cooked animal protein (ie ground turkey, beef, chicken)

Directions:

- Heat oven to 375 F. For silicone pan, spray with nonstick spray or coconut oil.
- Mix eggs in large bowl with seasonings, set aside.
- Sautee or blanch veggies and onions in a pan.
- Cook protein (ie turkey, chicken, beef, etc.).
- In the bottom of the muffin cups layer the following:
- Mix meat, vegetables, and onions. Fill muffin cups to be about 2/3 full, so that there is just enough room to add egg around the other ingredients.
- Use silicone, paper-liners, or regular muffin tins – simply spray with coconut oil or other baking spray first.
- Pour egg mix into each muffin cup until it is 3/4 full. Stir gently with a fork.
- Bake 25-35 minutes until muffins have risen, slightly browned, and set.

Muffins will keep more than a week in the refrigerator. These are great for kid's lunches.

Sun Dried Tomato Meatballs with Creamy Pesto

This is a delicious way to pack some healthy protein for you and your kids! It's also fun to dish up and eat (on sticks) and loaded with healthful spices and herbs. Enjoy knowing your children are getting their garlic, basil, pink salt, and coconut oil in one meal!

- 2 lbs ground Bison (great source of omega 3 fatty Acids!
- 2 tbsp chives minced
- 2 tbsp fresh basil minced
- ½ c minced sun dried tomatoes packed in olive oil
- 2 -3 garlic cloves minced
- 1 tsp pink Himalayan sea salt
- 1 tsp black pepper
- 1 tbsp coconut oil

Creamy Pesto:

- 1 c walnuts, halved or chopped
- ½ c extra virgin olive oil
- 3 garlic cloves
- ½ teaspoon pink Himalayan sea salt
- 2 c fresh basil leaves
- ¼ c sun dried tomatoes
- ½ c coconut cream (Overnight, chill a 13.5oz can of full fat coconut milk ie: Thai Kitchen brand. The cream on top will solidify-- scoop out ½ c of this coconut cream).

Directions:

- Preheat oven to 375.
- Combine all of the meatball ingredients together (EXCEPT the coconut oil) and shape into meatballs – golf ball sized.

- Heat skillet over medium/medium-high heat and add the tbsp of coconut oil. When oil is melted and skillet is hot, add the meatballs. Brown the meatballs on all sides.
- If you're using an oven safe skillet, cover it, place it in the oven, and cook for another 7-10 minutes. If you're not using an oven safe skillet, move the meatballs to a baking dish, cover and then oven cook for 7-10 minutes.
- Prepare pesto as meatballs cook – with the below directions.
- In food processor or blender combine: walnuts, olives, garlic, and salt. Process until smooth textured.
- Combine remaining pesto ingredients and process/blend again until smooth. Coconut cream adds a delicious creaminess to this pesto that you and your family will love!

Super Celery Juice

This juice is packed with both nutrient dense foods and kid-friendly flavors! Try this one out to get your kids green on the inside, clean on the inside!

- 1 apple
- 3 leaves kale
- ½ cucumber (large)
- 3 stalks celery

The New Lean "Happier Meal" Chicken Nuggets

As kids, we used to shake in anticipation at the fast food drive-through. The scent of fried grease could be smelled two blocks away and it seemed like heaven. Since those days, we've upgraded! So, we decided to hook you up with a favorite drive-through snack, redone with YOUR kids in mind.

- 24-ounce chicken breast cutlets
- 1 cup of coconut flour
- ½ cup of chopped almonds (or walnuts)
- 2 tablespoons of coconut oil
- 3 large organic eggs – beaten
- 1 teaspoon of cayenne pepper
- 1/4 teaspoon of paprika
- 1 teaspoon of garlic powder
- 1 tablespoon of pink salt

Healthy Options:

Go Free-Range Organic: Current practices of chicken farming can be harmful to our bodies by increasing the incidents of antibiotics in the poultry. Since we then eat and absorb these chemicals, it is vital to buy chicken that is raised "free-range," or chickens that were free to forage through open fields to eat seeds, grains, vegetation, worms and insects. The levels of natural Omega-3 are much greater in free-range organic chicken while also providing a unique and desirable flavor.

Get the Crunch with Almonds: An easy trick to enhance the crunch and flavor of your nuggets is to go with chopped almonds. Simply chop up ½ cup of almonds (or walnuts) for a great crunch kids are sure to enjoy! Add this to the "breading" mixture.

Ever Heard of Coconut Flour? Critical for baking, bleached flour is often devoid of nutrients and can cause gastrointestinal disrepair. We discovered a unique product made of one of the healthiest foods on earth – coconut. Coconut flour is gluten-free and 58% fiber, making it a perfect choice for our chicken coating.

Directions:

- Whisk eggs in medium-sized bowl, dip chicken cutlets in coconut flour (set aside in small bowl) and set floured chicken cutlets in beaten egg mixture.
- In a shallow bowl combine: coconut flour, chopped almonds, paprika, garlic powder, Italian seasoning, cayenne, and pink salt. Use a spatula to combine ingredients. Gather mixture and spread evenly over a cookie sheet lined with paper towels. This is your "breading" mixture.
- Begin heating coconut oil in a large skillet turned to medium heat.
- Remove chicken from egg mixture, allowing excess liquid to drain. Place chicken cutlets on "breading" mixture, evenly spreading to coat both sides.
- Place chicken cutlets in heated coconut oil until they are golden and crispy (about five minutes per side). When done, allow chicken to cool and serve with a side of fresh veggies (ie steamed broccoli) and a little Dijon mustard or tomato paste for flavor.

Not Your Normal Nachos

What kid doesn't LOVE nachos? Fortunately for you Fitlife Parents, Mexican food can easily be altered into a high-protein, allergen-free cuisine. This is one of our classic go-to meals that can be prepared in less than 10 minutes.

- Choose flax crackers, rice crackers or lettuce wedges
- 12 ounces of ground turkey meat
- 1 large tomato - diced
- 1 large red bell pepper – diced
- 1/2 cup green onions – minced
- 2 jalapeno peppers – minced
- 1 medium avocado – cubed
- Sriracha sauce to season
- Olive oil spray
- 1 teaspoon pink salt
- 1 teaspoon freshly ground black pepper

Healthy Options:

* Flax seed crackers: A great, high-fiber, crunchy, nutritious and tasty snack, loaded with Omega-3 fatty acids. These are great for improving brain function and are packed high in fiber.

* Rice crackers: These are just as crunchy and delicious and contain no gluten for people sensitive to high-gluten foods.

* Lettuce wedges: The classic nacho chip is loaded with sodium, contains empty calories, and often made with gluten. Try adding a combination of iceberg, green-leaf, and red-leaf lettuce for added presentation and nutrition.

* Go Turkey or Go Home: Turkey is a great, healthy option. Topping your nachos with turkey will provide kids with extended energy due to the higher protein content.
* Spice It Up: Sriracha is not only healthy, it's packed with delicious flavor too! *Note: if you've got a picky eater at home, test out the sriracha sauce with a small serving.
* Healthy Cheese Alternative: We know kids love cheese, so when trying to eliminate dairy (or minimize it) sprinkle Nutritional Yeast. This is loaded with B vitamins!

Directions:

– Preheat oven to 350° Fahrenheit.
– Place 12 ounces of ground turkey in a medium frying pan coated with olive oil spray. Using a spatula, separate turkey into smaller clumps. Add the salt and pepper and the desired amount of Sriracha to taste (about 1 tablespoon). Cook for 5 to 8 minutes or until done.
– Dice your raw vegetables into equally sized pieces: onion, tomato, green pepper, jalapeno, and avocado. If using lettuce, chop head into chip-sized pieces.
– Time Saver: Wash all of your vegetables and dice them up while the turkey is cooking.
– Oven should be preheated to 350° F. Line a baking sheet with aluminum foil and spray with olive oil spray. Spread the chips (if using) in a single layer on the foil. Distribute the seasoned turkey burger over the chips (if using chips or crackers and not lettuce). Sprinkle the cheese choice lightly on top of the chips. Bake in the

oven until the cheese is melted and the chips are warm (2 to 3 minutes).

- Remove the nachos from the oven and place onto serving plates. Sprinkle the raw tomatoes, bell pepper, green onions, and jalapenos on top of chips or lettuce. Add fresh-diced avocado chunks to top. Add one additional pinch of salt and any fresh herbs you see fit!

Guacamole eggs

This is a super fun snack option for kids and you! Plus, it's an amazing way to enjoy the benefits of eggs, some of which include improvements to eye function due to potent amounts of carotenoids, luteins, and zeaxanthins.

- 12 eggs, hard boiled
- 2 ripe avocados
- ½ onion, chopped small
- 2 tsp sea salt
- 2 tsp pepper

Directions:

- Peel and cut hard boiled eggs in half (the long way) and remove yolks with a spoon.
- *Note: do this carefully to preserve the outer egg white "cup" – we'll be filling each half with mixed ingredients.
- In a bowl, mix 6 egg yolks and avocado (should look similar to guacamole!).
- *Note: the other 6 yolks can be stored for later use or tossed.
- Add chopped onion, salt and pepper.

- Mix completely. Option: Add a small squeeze of lemon to preserve the green color!
- With a spoon, fill each egg white half with avocado mixture.

Jicama Chips & Guacamole Dip

Kids will love and enjoy this healthy FitLife upgrade for chips and guacamole! Ditch the chips and let your kids still enjoy the health benefits of avocados. They offer an amazing source of glutathione, which is the king of antioxidants.

- 1 large Jicama
- 1-2 Ripe avocados
- ¼ cup Onion diced small
- 1 tsp Pepper & 2 tsp Sea Salt

Directions:

- Slice jicama into quarters, then into thin, chip-like pieces.
- In a bowl, mix: avocado, onion, and seasonings.

Sweet Potato Rounds

Sweet potatoes are a great source of Beta carotene. They also pack more potassium than a banana but are also lower-glycemic than a regular potato. This means that your kid's blood sugar will not skyrocket and have them bouncing off the walls.

- 2 medium sweet potatoes – sliced into 1/4" thick rounds
- 1-1/2 tablespoon of coconut oil

- 1 tablespoon of cinnamon
- 2 tablespoons of raw honey (if desired)
- Pink salt and freshly ground black pepper to taste

Healthy Option:

Cinnamon for Flavor and Health: This sweet spice is rich in antioxidants and also controls blood sugar. Just a small amount has been known to reduce blood sugar in Type 2 Diabetics and lower triglycerides and LDL cholesterol. It's a unique and appetizing flavor to add to the texture of the sweet potatoes.

Directions:

- Preheat oven to 400° Fahrenheit.
- Toss sweet potato rounds, coconut oil, cinnamon, salt, and pepper in a large casserole, making sure to spread ingredients across entire surface of casserole.
- Bake for 20 minutes.
- If desired, at minute 17, drizzle on two tablespoons of raw honey. After two minutes of cooling, serve sweet potato rounds immediately.

"Cheesy" Fitlife Popcorn

Whether you pop your own or buy it from the store, you know how much kids enjoy popcorn! We've got a FitLife approved version for your family to try. It's simple and ultra tasty!

- ½ - ⅔ cup nutritional yeast
- ¼ cup olive oil
- 2 tsp sea salt
- 2 tsp pepper

Directions:

- Pop plain popcorn.
- Mix all ingredients in a large bowl and enjoy with the kids!

Option: Substitute Spirulina or greens powder for Yeast = Green super food popcorn!

Dairy Free Tapioca Pudding

This is a delicious Fitlife approved healthy alternative for tapioca pudding! We love that it's dairy free, and it's kid-tested to taste amazing.

- ½ cup full fat coconut milk
- 1 tbsp chia seeds
- 1 tbsp cinnamon
- 1 tsp sea salt
- Option: add cocoa powder to make it chocolate pudding!

Directions:

- Mix chia seeds and coconut milk.
- Let seeds expand for at least 30 minutes.
- Mix all the ingredients with a spoon or blender.

Surprise Kale Two Ways

We hope you've already tried and enjoyed our Fitlife kale chips—because we're here to tell you they can be even better! Here are two variations that we know your kids will love and ask for again and again.

1. Chocolate & Coconut Kale Chips

- 1 bunch of kale. Wash and remove stems.
- ½ cup cashews, soaked for 4-6hrs
- ¼ cup agave/honey (one or a combo)
- ⅓ cup cocoa powder
- 1 tsp vanilla extract
- ½ tsp cinnamon
- ¼ cup coconut flakes (unsweetened or sweetened)
- 2 tbsp coconut oil

Directions:

- Preheat oven to 300F.
- Soak cashews in water.
- Strain water from cashews; add all ingredients, except the kale, to a blender or VitaMix.
- Blend until smooth for chocolate coconut coating.
- Pour mix over bowl of washed, de-stemmed kale leaves and toss to coat.
- Add kale to parchment-lined baking sheet and bake at 300F for 20 minutes. Flip, and bake for roughly another 10 minutes.

**Watch them closely because the honey/agave/ mixture can burn easily! Your nose should help you determine how done these chips are!

2. "Cheesy" Kale Chips

- 1 large bunch of kale. Wash and remove stems.
- ½ cup Cashews
- ¼ cup olive oil (maybe less)

- 2 tsp sea salt
- 2 tsp pepper
- ¼ cup nutritional yeast

Directions:

- Preheat Oven to 350F.
- Chop kale leaves into small "bite-sized" pieces and set aside.
- With ¼ -1 cup water, blend cashews and nutritional yeast. Adjust water for desired consistency. We want this mixture to be able to coat the kale leaves.
- In a large mixing bowl, add olive oil, sea salt, and pepper.
- Add kale and cashew/yeast mixture.
- Spread onto a large baking sheet.
- Bake for 10-15 minutes – checking frequently!

FitLife Approved Parent's Grocery List

Produce

Apples, Avocados, Bananas, Bell Peppers, Blackberries, Blueberries, Carrots, Celery, Cucumbers, Golden Beets, Jicama, Kale, Lettuce, Spinach, Strawberries, Sweet Potatoes

Protein

Chicken Breast, Eggs, Ground Turkey or Beef, Protein Powder (vanilla or chocolate)

Seasonings

Cayenne Pepper, Cinnamon, Garlic Powder, Paprika, Pepper, Sea Salt, Sriracha Sauce,
Vanilla Extract

Super Foods/Other

Almond Milk/Coconut Milk (unsweetened), Chia Seeds, Cocoa Powder, Coconut Flour, Flax Crackers (or substitute Jicama, Rice Crackers, Lettuce Wedges, etc.), Nutritional Yeast, Popcorn, Raw Honey

Healthy Fats

Almonds, Almond Butter, Canned Coconut Milk (Thai Kitchen), Cashews, Coconut Flakes, Coconut Oil, Olive Oil

This Is Just The Beginning…Of Their Lives

If you enjoyed this book, share it with your children. Read it with them and get them excited about making healthy choices.

It will be the best investment you ever make, in your children's health

Speaking of investments, I invite you to check out my other bestselling books about health, juicing and trimming your belly, available on Amazon now

Now Get These Other Bestselling Books By Drew Canole on Amazon Too:

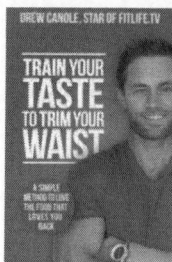

Train Your Taste To Trim Your Waist
http://amzn.to/1GEdKmr

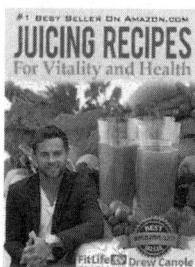

Juicing Recipes for Vitality & Health
http://amzn.to/1GEdXX1

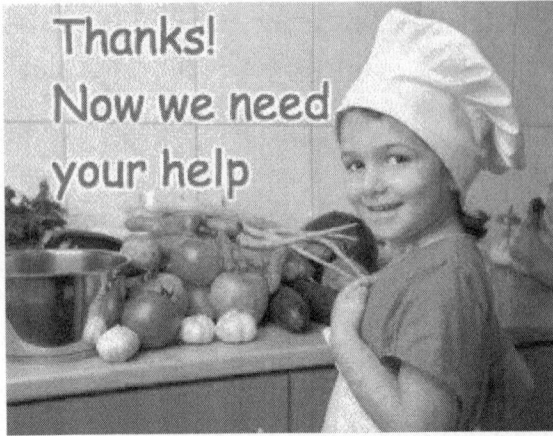

Thanks!
Now we need
your help

Thank you for reading Drew's book.
More kids need to read it and parents need to know
how good it is.

Please REVIEW this book on Amazon. Drew needs
your feedback and readers need to know if you
recommend it as a good investment (or not)

About the Author

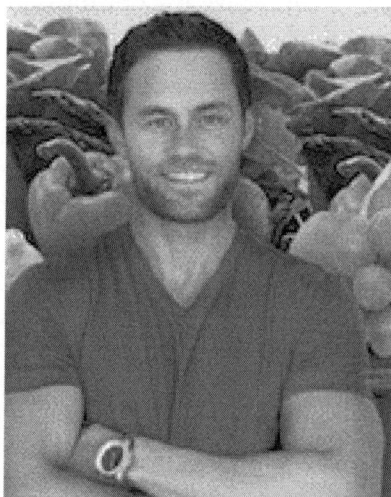

Drew Canole, bestselling author and transformation specialist is the nation's leading evangelist for the healing and transformative power of juicing vegetables and fruits.

Thousands of fans, clients, moms and dads have followed Drew's advice and introduced juicing into their lives, witnessing amazing results in their waist size, energy levels and overall health.

Now as a follow up to the bestselling "Juicing Recipes for Vitality & Health" book and the critically acclaimed "Train Your Taste To Trim Your Waist" Drew brings you his guide and recipe book designed specifically for parents and their kids.

From The Kitchen Of Drew Canole

For the past several years my readers, fans and clients have sent me story after story about how juicing vegetables and eating whole foods has changed, sometimes even saved, their lives. Since I read each and every testimonial, I started noticing a trend. Parents were writing in about their children. Their emails either asked me how to get their children "on the juice" or extolling the benefits their children have been receiving by replacing soft drinks with green drinks.

Stories flooded in about how juicing either reduced or eliminated their children's ADD/ADHD symptoms or restored their energy and their health. Some reported cases of acne disappearing and other seeming miraculous benefits. But if you understand how and why juicing works so well, you'll realize it's not miraculous at all, it simply restores us to the way nature intended us to be: healthy and vibrant.

Inspired by these stories, questions and suggestions, I sat down with my team at the Fitlife Kitchen and created a brand new book designed to give parents and children a fun, resourceful method to get into juicing for vitality and health.

This was the most fun book that I've ever written, because as I was writing I became excited with the idea that I was helping to "juice up" the next generation.

If this book helps keep just one child from ruining their health with sugary soft drinks and turns them onto a lifetime of positive nutrition choices, then it's worth all of the work it's taken to bring this book to you.

They say it takes a village to raise a child…and I believe it. That's why you'll always hear me say…

We're in this together,
Drew Canole
Fitlife.tv

Join us on Facebook.com/vegetablejuicing

9260078R00071

Printed in Great Britain
by Amazon.co.uk, Ltd.,
Marston Gate.